Drug Abuse and Society™

STEROIDS
HIGH-RISK PERFORMANCE DRUGS

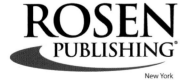

ROSEN
PUBLISHING®

New York

Jeri Freedman

To my niece and nephew, Laura and Matthew Freedman, with love

Published in 2009 by The Rosen Publishing Group, Inc.
29 East 21st Street, New York, NY 10010

First Edition

Library of Congress Cataloging-in-Publication Data

Freedman, Jeri.
Steroids: high-risk performance drugs / Jeri Freedman.—1st ed.
    p. cm.—(Drug abuse and society)
Includes bibliographical references and index.
ISBN-13: 978-1-4358-5013-2 (library binding)
1. Steroid abuse. 2. Steroids—Social aspects. 3. Steroids—Physiological effects. 4. Steroids—Metabolism. 5. Doping in sports. I. Title.
HV5822.S68F74 2009
613.8—dc22

                                        2008013413

Manufactured in Malaysia

Contents

INTRODUCTION

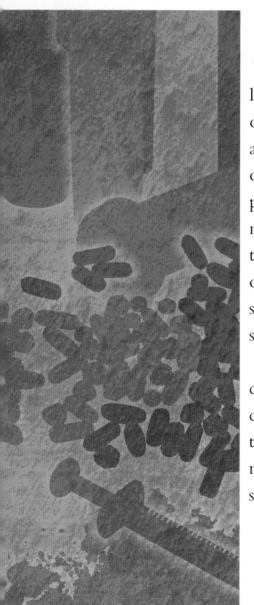

Steroids are powerful drugs that affect many parts of your body. Steroid use has been a hot topic in the media lately. You may have heard or read that some of the biggest names in sports have been accused of using steroids. Steroids, which on the street are also known as stackers, pumpers, gym candy, weight trainers, and, most commonly, juice, seem to be all over the place. Everywhere experts are arguing over the effects of steroid use on individuals, sports, and society. What exactly are steroids, though?

Steroids are similar to hormones, the chemicals produced in the human body that control its metabolism (the processes that take place in the body). The steroids that are most often abused are those based on male sex hormones, such as testosterone, which

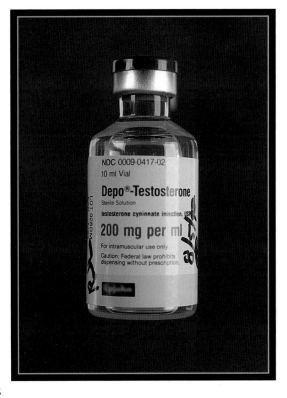

Depo-Testosterone, pictured here, is an example of an injectable steroid intended for medical use only, with a prescription. It is used to treat men with low testosterone levels and some cancers.

are produced primarily in the testes. These steroids are responsible for the development of male characteristics, such as facial hair and large muscles. This type of steroid is called an anabolic steroid. Anabolic steroids build up muscle tissue, making muscles bigger and stronger.

Today, most steroids used for medical purposes are synthesized, or made, in laboratories. These steroids are used medically to treat a wide variety of diseases, including muscle wasting, growth deficiency, asthma, skin conditions, and others.

Synthetic steroids are used not only medically but also illegally for bodybuilding purposes by people participating in sports or combat. Two groups of people commonly abuse steroids: athletes who feel that building up more muscle will give them a competitive edge and people who are concerned with their personal attractiveness, who feel that building up muscle will enhance their physique. These athletes may be people who are looking for a shortcut, to avoid the hard work necessary to build up muscles by working out. Or, they may lack confidence in their own abilities and believe that they won't be able to win without artificial aid. The second group of people who abuse steroids includes teenagers who believe that a leaner, more muscular body will make them more attractive to the opposite sex.

Steroids are often used by doctors to treat certain types of medical problems and, therefore, are available legally only with a prescription. Steroids can be obtained in the form of pills, creams, and injectable liquids. The forms most commonly abused are the pills and injectable liquids. When people illegally use steroids, they often take ten to sixty times the amount prescribed for medical treatment.

Buying and using steroids without a prescription is illegal. It is also dangerous. Steroids have many serious effects on the body and mind. Too much of them can cause harm and permanent damage.

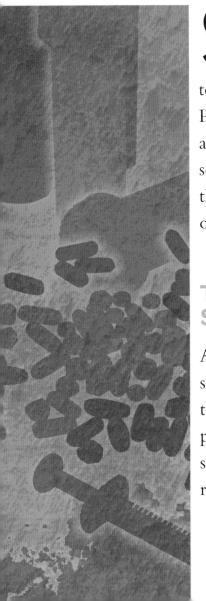

CHAPTER 1
The Nature of Steroids

Steroid abuse scandals in the past few years have included football and baseball players, professional wrestlers, teenaged basketball players, and rap artists. People hear so much about the use and abuse of steroids in the news today that it seems to be a fairly recent problem. In fact, the use—and abuse—of steroids throughout the world go back a long way.

THE DISCOVERY OF STEROIDS

Arnold Berthold (1803–1861), a German scientist, was the first person to demonstrate that a substance produced in the testes played a role in the development of male sexual characteristics. He observed that when rooster testes were transplanted into the abdomen of roosters from whom they had been removed, the roosters developed normal male characteristics. This showed that they contained a substance that was responsible for the development of male features.

Interest in the powers of male steroids was advanced by experiments performed by Charles Édouard Brown-Séquard (1817–1894), a French doctor, in the 1880s. Brown-Séquard injected himself with an extract from the testes of guinea pigs and dogs. In 1889, he reported to the scientific community in Paris that these extracts increased his strength and alertness. As a result, physicians began giving patients injections of the extracts, and makers of patent medicines began including such extracts in their products. In 1920, Eugen Steinach (1861–1944), an Austrian scientist, developed a surgical operation designed to increase the output of testosterone from the testes. It became popular in the first half of the twentieth

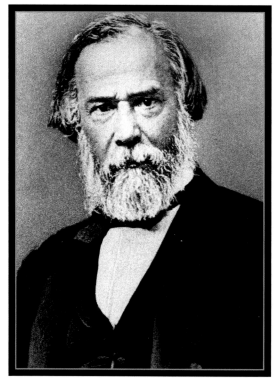

Charles Édouard Brown-Séquard was a nineteenth-century French doctor who popularized the use of male hormones to increase the strength and vitality of men.

century among middle-aged men, who believed that it made them feel younger and more energetic.

The first male steroid isolated and identified by scientists was androsterone. It was isolated by German chemist Adolf Butenandt (1903–1995) in 1931. The pharmaceutical industry was greatly interested in being able to supply steroids to the public because of the popular interest in their rejuvenating qualities. "Rejuvenating" means that they made people feel younger. Once such a chemical was identified, it did not take long for scientists to create it in their labs. In 1934, Leopold Ruzicka (1887–1976), a Swiss chemist, started making androsterone. Then, in 1935, four chemists at the Organon Company in the Netherlands isolated an even stronger male hormone from the testes—testosterone. Later that same year, testosterone was already being manufactured by the Schering Corporation. In 1939, Butenandt and Ruzicka were awarded the Nobel Prize for Chemistry for their discoveries; however, the Nazi government of Germany made Butenandt decline his award.

HISTORY OF PERFORMANCE-ENHANCING DRUG USE

People have been consuming performance-enhancing substances for many centuries. In ancient Greece, athletes consumed items such as sesame seeds, certain potions, and large quantities of meat, which they believed would improve their physical abilities. Fred Lorz, the man who won the gold medal in the marathon in the Olympics in 1904, drank a mixture of the chemical strychnine in brandy before his race because he believed it would improve his performance. At the end of the race, it knocked him out.

Performance-enhancing drug use became a widespread problem in the years just after World War II (1939–1945). In the late 1930s and early 1940s, a class of drugs called amphetamines was developed. Amphetamines are stimulants, which make people feel as if they have more energy. Athletes promptly started using them because they believed the drugs improved their athletic performance.

It did not take long for the discovery of steroids to affect the sports scene. As word of the energizing and strength-enhancing effects of steroids spread, they became the drugs of choice. Extensive use of steroids began in weight lifting, where there is an obvious advantage to having big, strong muscles. The Soviet Union was the first country to give its weight lifters steroids in the 1950s. But by the mid-1960s, steroids were being used by Olympic weight lifters from a number of other countries, including the United States. The use of steroids spread from weight lifters to other types of athletes who wanted a so-called edge. By the end of the 1960s, the use of steroids was so widespread that the International Olympic Committee started testing athletes for use of steroids and banning them if they found evidence of the practice. The most famous use of steroids in sports is probably that by the women on the East German Olympic teams, including

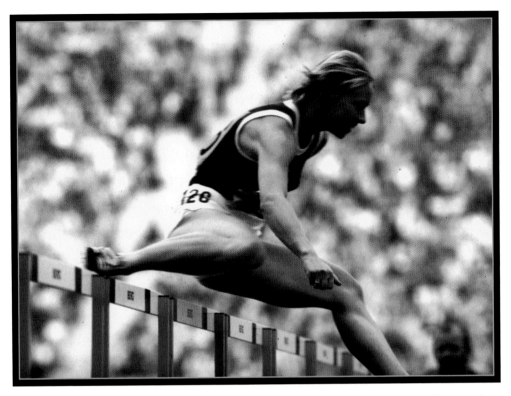

Annelie Erhardt of East Germany competes in the 100-meter hurdles at the 1972 Summer Olympics. The East German track team's coaches were later found to have given the athletes steroids to improve their performances.

track and field, swimming, and canoeing, in the 1970s. In 1972, East Germany won forty medals. In 1976, that number jumped to ninety, and in 1980 to one hundred twenty-six. It was later revealed that the coaches had been doping their athletes, including some girls as young as twelve and thirteen, with steroids and without the athletes' knowledge. A number of women on the team later suffered from a variety of physical side effects such as ovarian cysts, inflammation, and unwanted body hair.

In 1990, steroids were added to the Controlled Substances Act by the U.S. government. The Controlled Substances Act regulates the manufacturing, importing, distribution, and possession of drugs. It identifies various types of potentially dangerous drugs, and it provides appropriate penalties for illegally producing, selling, and using them.

From the last few decades of the twentieth century to the present day, there has been a constant stream of scandals involving the use of steroids to enhance performance in college and professional sports.

WHAT STEROIDS NATURALLY DO IN THE BODY

The anabolic steroids that are used to enhance performance are male sex hormones, primarily testosterone. Small amounts of testosterone are produced by the adrenal glands (small glands that sit on the kidneys). The majority of testosterone is produced in the testes. It is responsible for the development of male characteristics such as facial hair, thick muscles, and the ability to produce sperm. A small amount of testosterone is also produced in the ovaries of women because women need some testosterone for activities such as healthy bone growth. However, too much

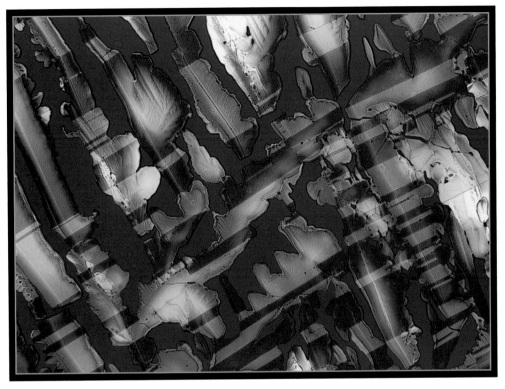

This image, which was taken through a microscope using polarized light, shows the crystals that make up the male sex hormone testosterone. Testosterone is an androgen, a steroid hormone, that is responsible for the development of male reproductive organs and masculine characteristics.

testosterone will cause masculinization (the development of male physical characteristics) in women. That is what happened to the East German female Olympic athletes in the 1970s. Some were required to undergo gender-verification tests to prove that they were not men in disguise!

13

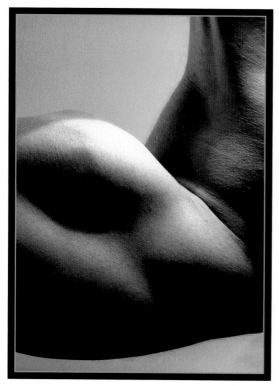

Abusing testosterone can cause an abnormal growth of muscle tissue, leading to limited mobility.

HOW STEROIDS WORK

Steroids cause a person to develop muscle by increasing the rate at which protein (the building block of muscle) is produced in the body. One way that anabolic steroids increase muscle size is by prompting the body to make more muscle tissue. Another way in which they lead to abnormally large muscles is by blocking the action of a chemical in the body called cortisol. When people experience stress, the body releases cortisol, which produces various changes in the body that make it able to run faster or fight harder. This performance boost gives people a better chance of survival when they're facing a physical threat. However, strenuous exercise also leads to the release of cortisol, and one of the side effects of cortisol is that it breaks down tissue. One of the effects of anabolic steroids is to block the activity of cortisol so that tissue is not broken down. Because they block cortisol, these steroids cause one to build up more muscle tissue than normal and to break down less. As a result, people who abuse anabolic steroids can develop very large muscles, a condition called hypertrophy.

Teen Steroid Abuse Statistics

For the 2007 Monitoring the Future study on teen drug abuse, which was conducted by the National Institute on Drug Abuse and the University of Michigan, researchers surveyed for steroid abuse 16,495 eighth graders in 151 schools, 16,398 tenth graders in 120 schools, and 15,132 twelfth graders in 132 schools. (The samples are representative of students in the respective grades in public and private secondary schools across the United States.) They reported these results:

- 1.5 percent of eighth graders have used steroids.
- 1.8 percent of tenth graders have used steroids.
- 2.2 percent of twelfth graders have used steroids.

Dr. Carla Laos of the University of Florida Pediatric Program and Dr. Jordan D. Metzl of the Sports Medicine Institute for Young Athletes, Hospital of Special Surgery, coauthors of a 2006 article, "Performance-Enhancing Drug Use in Young Athletes," reported that surveys show the following:

- 30 percent of teenagers who have tried steroids are female.
- 25 percent of adult steroid users began using in their teens.

MEDICAL USES OF STEROIDS

Steroids are used by prescription to treat certain types of medical disorders. They are used to treat boys and men who don't produce enough male hormones for normal development. For example, they are given to men who have testes removed because of testicular cancer and in treatments for impaired growth. They are also used to treat some forms of anemia (a condition in which a person has too few red blood cells), certain types of cancers, autoimmune diseases, certain skin diseases, and osteoporosis (the loss of bone, which often occurs as people age). In addition, researchers are currently investigating the application of steroids in encouraging tissue growth after major surgery and for treating burn victims.

WHY DO YOUNG PEOPLE USE STEROIDS?

Teenagers are often self-conscious, unsure of their attractiveness, and dissatisfied with their bodies. At the same time, they are deeply concerned about attracting potential dates or partners. These feelings of apprehension lead some teenagers to use steroids as a way of guaranteeing a leaner, more muscular body, which they believe will make them more attractive to others.

In sports, steroid use is even more widespread. One reason for this prevalence is that sports are no longer seen as a recreational activity or a chance to spotlight one's natural talent. Now that athletes can be drafted onto professional sports teams while still in college, or even directly out of high school, playing sports is no longer about having fun; it's about making big money. The financial rewards have made winning a serious business. And many people will do whatever it takes to win.

CHAPTER 2

Abusing Steroids

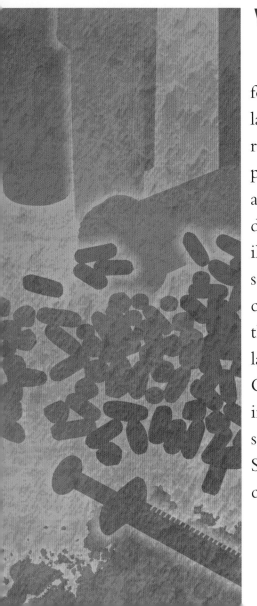

Widespread distribution of anabolic steroids is possible because synthetic (man-made) forms of the chemical can be produced in large quantities. However, such production requires the proper equipment, so the process is not cheap. Some illegal steroids are obtained from dishonest pharmacists, doctors, or veterinarians. However, most illegal steroids come from one of two sources: pharmaceutical or chemical companies that manufacture them outside the United States and Canada; or illegal laboratories within the United States and Canada. In the former case, drug dealers import the drugs from sources in places such as Bulgaria, the Czech Republic, Slovakia, Thailand, and Mexico. In the latter case, the drugs are made in secret laboratories

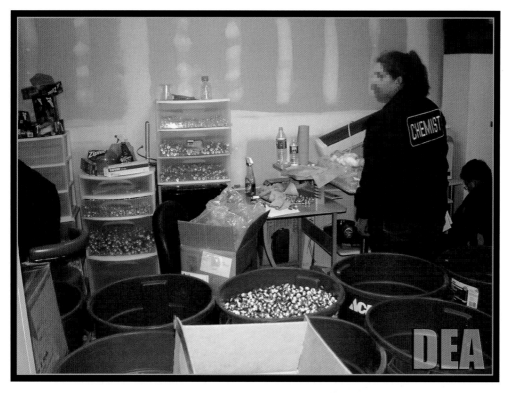

In September 2007, agents from the U.S. Drug Enforcement Administration (DEA) seized 11.4 million units of steroids in an international investigation called Operation Raw Deal. The investigation included the seizure of fifty-six laboratories that were making steroids across the United States.

and then sold on the street. Both sources of illegal steroids have considerable health risks. There are no controls on how the products are made, and they may well be contaminated. There is also the risk that, like other illegal drugs, the products have been "cut" (or diluted) with some other substance to make them go further when sold on the street. In addition, some illegal steroids are chemically altered so that their effects last longer in the body.

These modifications can increase their effects (and dangerous side effects), particularly when large doses are taken regularly.

Like other illegal drugs, steroids are sold to users by a network of dealers. Most often, these dealers sell to athletes at gyms, in locker rooms, and at athletic competitions. There are also many dealers who offer to sell steroids via the mail. Often, they approach potential buyers via e-mail or sites on the Internet, sometimes claiming to be overseas pharmacies or chemical supply houses. Many of these sources, however, actually supply fake steroids. Because you are purchasing an illegal product, you have no way to get your money back when you are cheated.

USING STEROIDS

Athletes who illegally use steroids increase the total amount of steroids in their body beyond the normal, healthy level provided by their naturally produced steroids. But the problem is not just adding a small amount of extra steroids. Athletes who use steroids generally take doses ten to sixty times as great as those given for medical purposes. Taking a huge amount of substances such as steroids is called megadosing. Some steroid users gradually increase their dosage over a period of time until they reach a peak dose and then gradually decrease their dose over the same amount of time; this is called pyramiding. Some users engage in a process called cycling. They take varying amounts of steroids over

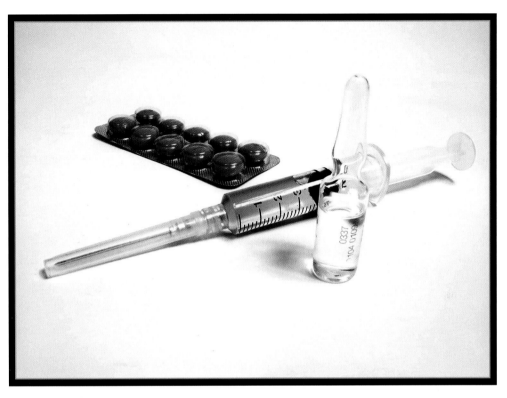

Two forms of steroids—pill and injectable (in vial)—are shown here with a syringe. "Stacking" steroids, by taking different forms at the same time, increases the chances of dangerous side effects.

a period of weeks, then stop taking them, and then start the cycle again. In addition, some steroid users both inject steroids and take steroid pills, or use steroids in combination with other performance-enhancing compounds, such as human growth hormone. This practice of taking several forms of steroids at the same time is called stacking. As with taking any combination of multiple drugs, this is a dangerous habit. The high dose of

21

Responding to Pressure to Use Steroids

Whenever you let your friends or teammates talk you into doing something you would not ordinarily do, you are giving in to peer pressure. Friends can be a valuable source of support and encouragement as you try new activities. Sometimes, however, your friends or teammates will try to influence your actions negatively, for example, by trying to get you to drink alcohol or use steroids. One reason for this behavior is that they don't really feel comfortable doing those things, or they know they're wrong. They feel that if they can get others to go along with them, they can justify their behavior. It's often hard for people to resist peer pressure because they fear being kicked out of the group and isolated. Also, if people don't go along, members of the group might put them down in front of others.

Even though it is difficult to stand up to peer pressure, there are times when it is important to do so. When you are pressured to do something illegal or harmful to your health, you need to protect yourself. As you are growing up, you have to make more and more decisions about what is right for you as an individual. If you feel uncomfortable about doing something, don't do it. Your mind is telling you it's wrong. If you participate in sports or other activities where it's likely that at some point someone may offer you steroids, plan in advance what you'll say. With the emphasis today on healthy living, it's perfectly natural to refuse to put artificial compounds in your body.

If you refuse to be pressured into doing negative things, you may be surprised to find that some of your peers are glad to follow your lead and refuse to participate as well. Many are just as uncertain as you are, but they lack the courage to stand up to peer pressure on their own.

steroids causes a major increase in all the activities controlled by anabolic steroids in the body and has far worse effects than just increasing muscle mass and athletic stamina.

PHYSICAL EFFECTS OF STEROID ABUSE

Common physical effects of steroid abuse include acne and the formation of striae—visible purplish ridges or furrows on the skin. Steroids can affect your heart and blood vessels. They can cause high blood pressure, an increase in the force required for the heart to force blood through the blood vessels. They increase the amount of low-density lipoprotein (LDL) cholesterol that your body produces. LDL cholesterol is a fatty substance that clogs your arteries, making it harder for blood to get through. The buildup of cholesterol on the walls of your arteries increases your

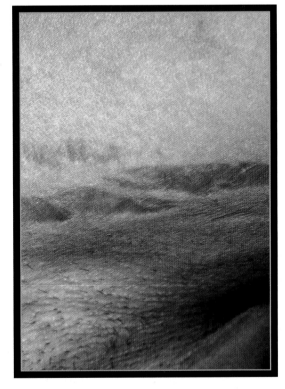

Striae are unattractive stretch marks that result from the thinning and loss of elasticity in the lower layer of the skin. Striae can be caused by steroid abuse.

chances of having a heart attack and stroke (the clogging of a blood vessel in the brain).

Abusing steroids can damage your liver and keep it from functioning normally, which is critical for purifying your blood, and it can also increase your chances of getting liver cancer. Steroids can damage your kidneys and cause you to get kidney stones, hard balls of minerals that cause great pain. They can also cause severe muscle cramps, especially in your abdomen and legs.

In addition, there are gender-related changes that take place in the body as a result of steroid abuse. Physical effects in males include impotence and an inability to make sperm, which can affect the ability to have children. If you are genetically prone

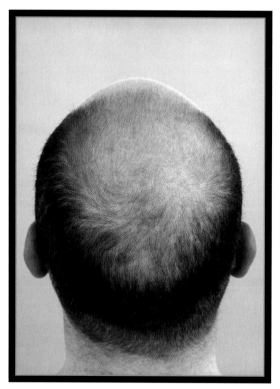

to male pattern baldness (that is, if older men in your family tend to go bald), then an increase in testosterone can cause you to start going bald, even though you're young. You may also experience the development of breasts.

If baldness runs in your family, abusing steroids can cause you to go bald—even if you're female and even if you're a teen.

This happens because your body starts to produce the female sex hormone estrogen to counteract the high levels of testosterone in your blood.

The effects of steroid abuse on women include masculinization, or male sex-related characteristics. In many ways, male hormones have the same effect on women as on men. They make the muscles large, but they also thicken the vocal cords, deepening a woman's voice. They also make facial hair grow and cause the breasts to shrink. Because getting one's period is controlled by the levels of various female hormones (such as estrogen) in the blood, an abnormally high level of male hormones and a proportionately lower level of female hormones can cause a woman's period to become irregular or stop altogether. They can also lead to difficulty in becoming pregnant and can result in birth defects.

The effects of steroids already mentioned are the same for teenagers and adults. Nevertheless, there are unique ways that steroids can affect teenagers. Steroids affect growth. Teenagers are still growing. Usually, people will not reach their full size until they are in their early twenties. How does your body know when to stop growing? It relies on the level of steroids in your blood. Therefore, if you take steroids, you can stunt your growth. When the level of anabolic steroids in your blood equals that present in an adult's blood, your body sees this as an indication that you are fully grown, even though you aren't. In addition, using steroids when you are a teenager can lead to permanent sterility (inability to have children).

PSYCHOLOGICAL EFFECTS OF STEROID ABUSE

Psychological effects are those that affect the mind. Abusing steroids affects your mood and behavior. Steroids affect a part of the brain called the hypothalamus. The hypothalamus is a region of the brain that helps regulate mood, body temperature, sleep, and food intake, among other things. Studies have shown that testosterone stimulates the part of the brain responsible for aggression and anger. Abusing steroids frequently causes mood swings—in which a person goes from being depressed (abnormally sad) to manic (abnormally frenzied and agitated). Steroid abuse often results in decreased sex drive. In addition, it can lead to increased feelings of rage and violent behavior.

CHAPTER 3
Coping with Steroid Abuse

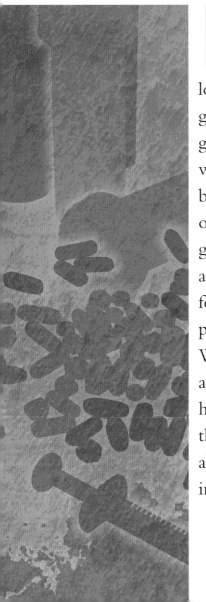

Mike was self-conscious. When he looked at himself in the locker-room mirror, he thought he looked scrawny compared to the other guys. He knew from watching TV that girls liked guys with muscles. Mike tried working out more, but he still lacked the big chest and arm muscles that the guys on TV always seemed to have. One of the guys at the gym told him about steroids and said he could get Mike some. Mike forked over one hundred dollars for some pills. He started taking several every day. When he used them up, he bought more and started taking more. On the Internet, he read about injectable steroids and how they were more powerful than using pills alone. Mike bought some syringes and injectable steroids. He was spending a big chunk of the money from his part-time job on steroids, but, as his muscles got bigger, he felt it was worth it.

By now, Mike was using both injectable steroids and pills several times each day. He decided to put his newfound strength to the test. He tried out for the baseball team and felt proud when he was chosen. As part of the screening process, he was required to get a physical. To his surprise, the doctor said that his blood pressure was abnormally high for someone his age. He asked Mike if he was taking any drugs, but Mike denied it. One day, Mike noticed that his hair seemed to be falling out when he brushed it, and his hairline was receding. He recognized the signs; his father was going bald—but his father was middle-aged, not a teenager. Some of the sites Mike had seen on the Internet had links that listed the side effects of steroids, but he had never paid any attention to them. He was sure nothing like that would ever happen to him. Now he was worried. Abruptly, without telling anyone, he decided to stop using steroids. He went from feeling pumped up to feeling dragged out. Everything now seemed miserable. He lost interest in baseball and schoolwork. He started to have thoughts about suicide. Mike's mother became increasingly worried about the moodiness of her usually easy-going son. She took Mike to a psychiatrist (a doctor who treats mental problems). The psychiatrist worked with Mike for almost a year to help him get over the depression from quitting steroids and his issues with his self-image. In the end, Mike was lucky—he wound up healthy and steroid-free. A lot of young people aren't that lucky. Many commit suicide or suffer serious health problems as a result of steroid abuse.

WHY PEOPLE BECOME ADDICTED

There is significant evidence that steroids are addictive. One reason that steroids are addictive is physiological—your body requires a certain amount of steroid hormones to function correctly. The body contains feedback systems to make sure that the proper level of a hormone is present. Chemical sensors in the body send a signal to the brain when the level of a hormone becomes too high or too low. The brain responds by sending a signal to the gland responsible for producing the hormone, telling it to make more or less. When you overload your system with anabolic steroids, the feedback system tells the brain that you have more than enough of these hormones in your body. Therefore, your body stops producing them. At that point, it becomes physically necessary for you to keep taking steroids from a source outside the body because the body is no longer capable of producing these hormones.

There is also a psychological aspect to steroid addiction. Many people take steroids in a deliberate attempt to improve their looks or athletic performance. Some athletes take them because they lack faith in their own abilities. Once they start to use

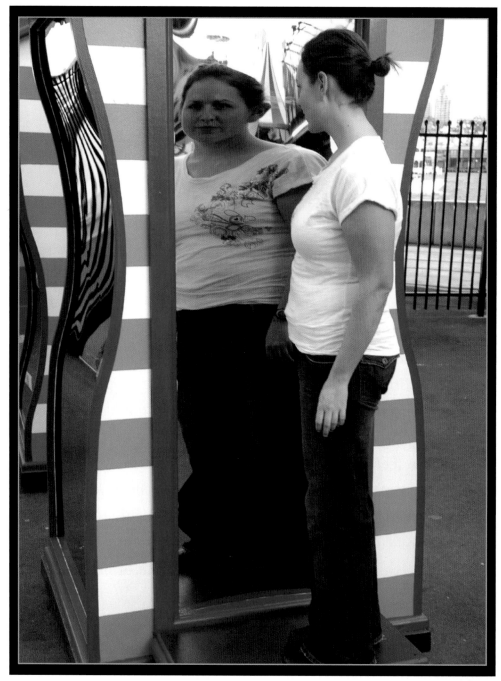

Many young people have a distorted impression of what their body looks like and how they appear to others. This condition is called dysmorphia or body dysmorphic disorder (BDD).

steroids, they become psychologically dependent on them. They don't believe they can perform well without them. Similarly, many young people take steroids because they believe that they will make them more attractive to the opposite sex. They see images of muscular men and women with sculpted bodies, and see the use of steroids as the way to develop that kind of body. Why do they keep using them? Because they don't believe they are attractive without them. This is a form of psychological, or mental, addiction. It can be further complicated by a distorted image of one's own body. Many young people who look perfectly fine believe that they are too fat or ugly in some way. They believe that it's necessary to change the way their body looks, and taking steroids is a way of doing that.

Signs of addiction are withdrawal symptoms, which occur when you stop taking the drug. In the case of steroids, if your body has shut down its own production of these compounds, the effects of removing the external source of steroids can be not only unpleasant but also dangerous.

IDENTIFYING STEROID ABUSE

One way in which steroid abuse is detected is by the observation of a doctor, teacher, coach, or anyone else who pays attention to students' behavior. Nowadays, many professionals such as these are on the lookout for signs of steroid abuse in students involved in sports like weight lifting, wrestling, and football, where such use

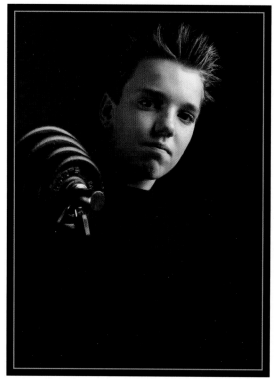

School staff members are on the lookout for telltale signs of steroid abuse, such as this twelve-year-old boy lifting a weight that is much too heavy for him.

could provide a significant advantage. One aspect they look for is telltale behavioral changes such as unusual aggression or depression. Another is frequent use of nutritional supplements, since athletes who use a lot of such supplements to enhance their performance often don't see any problem with using steroids. One reason for this increased watchfulness is that it's rare for a single athlete on a school team to be involved in steroid abuse. Usually, many team members are approached by the person who is supplying them with steroids. Even if a particular team member does not participate in the abuse, he or she often knows what's going on. If a student is caught using steroids, he or she often ends up providing the names of other users on the team because of threatened punishment or the offer of a reduced punishment. If you use steroids, there is a high likelihood that sooner or later you will be found out, either because someone notices your atypical behavior or because someone will turn you in.

A doctor may check for signs of steroid abuse as a part of a physical exam given to certify that the student is healthy enough either to start or to continue participation in sports. Key signs that a doctor looks for in males are shrinkage of the testicles, abnormal muscle development, and development of breast tissue. In females, some characteristics the doctor looks for are abnormal muscle development, facial hair, breast shrinkage, and baldness.

GETTING HELP

Some drug rehabilitation centers that treat drug addiction also handle steroid abuse. The names of such centers are usually available from your local hospitals and drug hotlines. Some people work with individual medical professionals instead of going for help at drug rehab centers. If you have been using steroids in large amounts or for a long period of time, it is especially important to talk with a medical professional. He or she can assist you in dealing with the physical and mental side effects and make sure that the level of steroids in your body is close to normal after you quit taking them. Those who want to stop abusing drugs often rely on the following three-pronged approach to treatment:

- Medical help to deal with the physical side effects when the drug is no longer taken
- Help from a mental health professional to deal with both the mental side effects from quitting and the underlying issues that led to the drug abuse
- Healthy exercise and nutrition to keep the body strong while withdrawing from the drug

Using this three-pronged approach increases the chance of a safe and healthy recovery because it treats the effects of withdrawal on your mind and body. As with any medical problem, the support of family and friends is also very important as a person goes through recovery.

Ten Great Questions to Ask a Doctor

1. Can you recommend a program to help me stop using steroids?
2. Is it OK to engage in physical activity while I'm experiencing withdrawal symptoms?
3. Do I need medication to help my body recover from steroid use?
4. What can I do about my feelings of depression?
5. What other performance-enhancing substances should I avoid?
6. What should I do if someone tries to get me to use steroids?
7. Has using steroids caused any problems with my body?
8. What treatment do you recommend for my physical problems?
9. Can you recommend a counselor I can talk to about my problem?
10. How can I build up my muscles without using steroids?

WITHDRAWAL SYMPTOMS

One of the difficulties of quitting the use of steroids is the severity of steroids' withdrawal symptoms. For this reason, if you have been using steroids and decide to quit, it is a good idea to seek professional help with managing the mental and physical symptoms. Physically, when you stop using steroids, your muscles will shrink and you may feel weaker. Mentally, you may suffer from depression (extreme feelings of sadness or hopelessness)

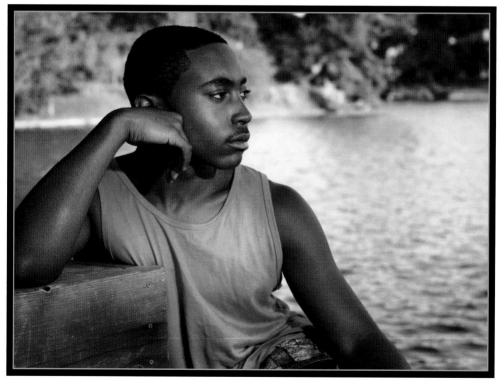

Withdrawing from steroids can lead to exaggerated feelings of hopelessness. You should seek help if you experience such feelings.

and lack of energy. It is especially important to realize that your depression is caused by the withdrawal from the steroids, and that your feelings are exaggerated. Mental health professionals can provide help in dealing with depression. It can take weeks or even months to recover from the effects of withdrawal, especially the mental effects such as depression.

Kicking the steroid habit usually requires a variety of approaches, including medical help with the physical symptoms of withdrawal, psychological help for depression, and social and behavioral training. This type of training is aimed at helping users develop a realistic body image and physical development and performance goals, as well as helping them deal with self-esteem issues.

CHAPTER 4
Steroid Use and the Law

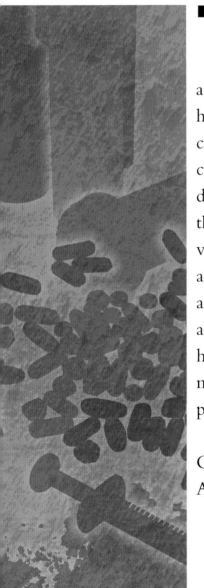

The Controlled Substances Act of 1990 was passed by the U.S. Congress to control the manufacture, distribution, and sale of certain drugs that are deemed harmful and likely to be abused. Drugs covered by the act are divided into classes, called schedules. Schedule I drugs are deemed to be the most dangerous and have the strongest regulations and penalties for violations. Anabolic steroids are categorized as Schedule III drugs. Schedule III drugs are considered to have less potential for abuse than Schedule I and II drugs and to have a legitimate medical use. They cause a moderate physical dependence and a high psychological (mental) dependence.

Congress first added steroids to the Controlled Substances Act in 1991. The Anabolic Steroid Control Act of 2004 was

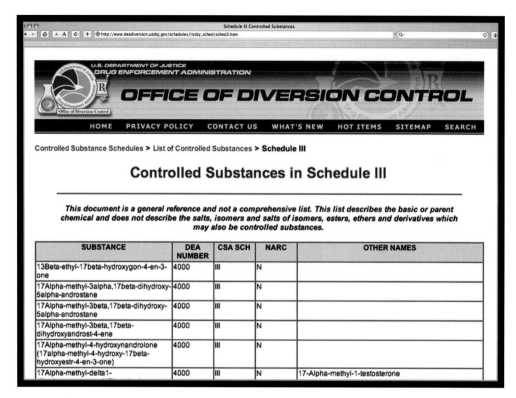

SUBSTANCE	DEA NUMBER	CSA SCH	NARC	OTHER NAMES
13Beta-ethyl-17beta-hydroxygon-4-en-3-one	4000	III	N	
17Alpha-methyl-3alpha,17beta-dihydroxy-5alpha-androstane	4000	III	N	
17Alpha-methyl-3beta,17beta-dihydroxy-5alpha-androstane	4000	III	N	
17Alpha-methyl-3beta,17beta-dihydroxyandrost-4-ene	4000	III	N	
17Alpha-methyl-4-hydroxynandrolone (17alpha-methyl-4-hydroxy-17beta-hydroxyestr-4-en-3-one)	4000	III	N	
17Alpha-methyl-delta1-	4000	III	N	17-Alpha-methyl-1-testosterone

The U.S. Drug Enforcement Administration (DEA) maintains a Web site (www.deadiversion.usdoj.gov) that lists the controlled substances in Schedule III of the Controlled Substances Act. The site also includes lists of controlled substances in alphabetical order, by schedule, or by chronological order by scheduling action, from 1970 to the present.

passed to include additional steroids on the list of banned substances and to increase the U.S. Drug Enforcement Administration's powers to regulate steroids and enforce laws against steroid abuse. Using steroids without a prescription is illegal. Manufacturing steroids is also illegal under this act. Selling steroids—or attempting to sell them—is a crime under the Controlled Substances Act as well, and doing so can result in large fines and up to five years in prison. Under the Anabolic Steroid Control Act of 2004, possession of illegal steroids is punishable by up to one year in jail for a first offense and up to two years if you have a prior conviction.

In addition to federal laws, many individual states have passed laws specially aimed at steroid usage among teenagers. Among the states that have done so are California, Florida, Iowa, Louisiana, Maine, Michigan, Minnesota, New Jersey, Pennsylvania, Texas, and Virginia. The laws cover a wide scope of issues, ranging from random drug testing for steroid use among high school athletes to twenty-year jail sentences for selling steroids to minors.

In Canada, steroids are regulated under the Controlled Drug and Substances Act. It is illegal to buy or sell them without a prescription. If you do so and are convicted, you can be sentenced to up to eighteen months in prison.

Be aware that law enforcement agents often monitor chat rooms and Web sites that sell steroids, so think twice before participating in an illegal purchase.

LEGAL RISKS OF STEROIDS

The risks from buying, selling, and using steroids aren't just health-related. If you get involved with illegal steroids, there are a number of ways in which you can run into trouble with law enforcement officers. As mentioned earlier, nowadays law enforcement officers monitor Internet chat sites and newsgroups. The U.S. Postal Service is on the lookout for illegal trafficking in steroids. Postal Service inspectors may open packages that come from addresses known for or suspected of distributing steroids. If they find illegal steroids, law enforcement agents may allow the package to be delivered and then arrest the recipient.

Limiting your buying to in-person purchases isn't protection, either. If law enforcement agents arrest someone for selling steroids, two actions can happen. First, that person could reveal the names of the people to whom he or she has sold steroids. Even if you are not arrested for buying or possessing a controlled substance, you will probably be banned from sports teams. Second, the police often let someone they have arrested continue to sell steroids, taking into custody those who purchase the drugs. Therefore, if you buy steroids from someone at school or sporting events, you could be putting yourself at risk legally and healthwise.

RULES AGAINST STEROID USE IN SPORTS

All major sports organizations have rules against using anabolic steroids. These include the National Basketball Association (NBA), National Football League (NFL), National Hockey League (NHL), and Major League Baseball (MLB). Despite these rules, there

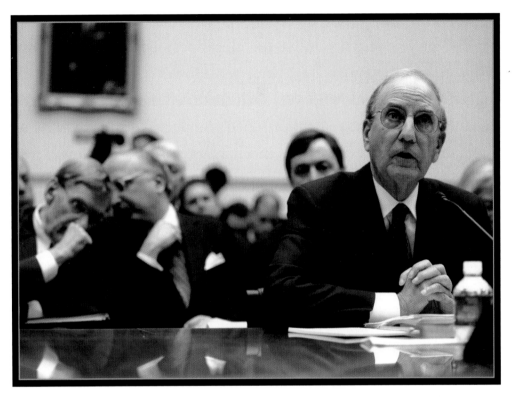

Former U.S. senator George Mitchell testifies at the U.S. House of Representatives committee hearing on the Mitchell Report, regarding the illegal use of steroids in Major League Baseball in 2008. Lawmakers warned baseball officials that tougher testing for the use of performance-enhancing drugs must be implemented in baseball by them or Congress would impose rules for the testing.

have been repeated scandals in recent years involving players in major league sports. One of the most significant events related to steroid use in professional sports was the release of the Mitchell Report in December 2007. Former U.S. senator George Mitchell undertook a twenty-month study of the use of anabolic steroids in professional baseball. According to the report, 5–7 percent of baseball players tested positive for illegal performance-enhancing drugs in an anonymous 2003 drug test. However, Senator Mitchell suggests that even more players than that used illegal performance-enhancing drugs such as steroids because players can take steps to normalize the level of steroids in their systems if they know when a drug test will take place. The players' union has consistently

Detecting Steroid Use

You've probably heard about athletes being asked to undergo drug testing for steroid use. How does a drug test actually work? The most common method of identifying steroids relies on a machine called a gas chromatograph. When you are given a drug test, you are asked to provide a urine sample in a small container. The chromatograph contains a central column packed with an absorbent material. A lab technician injects some of the sample into the column. The sample is gathered into the material in the column. An inert gas, like helium or argon, is blown through the column. It carries the molecules in the sample down a tube to a detector. The different types of molecules move down the tube at different rates. The detector can thus identify the different types of molecules in a sample. A computer then analyzes the results and indicates what type of compound would contain that combination of molecules. Gas chromatography works particularly well with artificial compounds such as laboratory-produced anabolic steroids because the combination of molecules they contain is well known. Therefore, it is easy to match the results from a urine sample to the known profile of a steroid.

fought the use of unannounced drug tests, which some people say further supports the idea that players are using anabolic steroids and don't want that fact found out. Because many players refused to be interviewed, it's impossible to know exactly how widespread the abuse is.

SPORTS STARS AND STEROID ABUSE

The Mitchell Report isn't the first major steroid investigation of the past decade. Throughout the 2000s, various investigations have revealed that there is a serious problem with professional athletes using steroids to enhance their performances. In 2003, the representatives of various U.S. government agencies that oversee the manufacture and distribution of controlled substances launched an investigation into the Bay Area Laboratory Co-Operative (BALCO). BALCO is a northern California company that provides blood and urine testing services and nutritional supplements to various clients, including well-known athletes. The government charged that the founder of the company, Victor Conte, had distributed a steroid disguised as a nutritional supplement to members of the NFL and MLB, and to certain Olympic athletes. Eventually, Conte pled guilty to illegal steroid distribution.

A number of athletes have admitted to illegal steroid use. One example is Paxton Clayton, who pitched for the Boston Red Sox in 2000 and 2001. He was released by the Red Sox in 2002 after getting a stress fracture in his back. He was later suspended from the Cincinnati Reds minor league team for violating the league's drug policy. In a June 22, 2006, article in *USA Today*, Clayton is quoted as saying, "I was taking way too much stuff [steroids], and I'd get rattled . . . You can't get rattled in the big leagues. And then I messed up my back. I think the steroids had something to do with that, too."

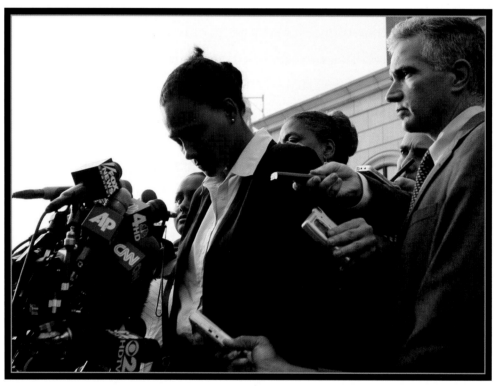

Track-and-field star Marion Jones talks to reporters after admitting to taking steroids in 2007. She said that she had broken trust with her fans and she was retiring from sports.

Another athlete who fell prey to the performance-enhancing drug habit is three-time Olympic gold medalist Marion Jones. In 2007, the track star admitted to having used steroids prior to the 2000 Olympic Games in Sydney, Australia. Not only did the International Olympic Committee strip her of the medals she won in the Olympics, but in January 2008, Jones was sentenced to six months in prison for lying to prosecutors about using steroids and participating in a scam to cash forged checks. In an article in the *International Herald Tribune*, U.S. District Court judge Kenneth Karas was quoted as saying that he sentenced Jones to prison time "to send a message to athletes who have abused drugs and overlooked the values of hard work, dedication, teamwork, and sportsmanship."

CHAPTER 5
Steroid Abuse and Society

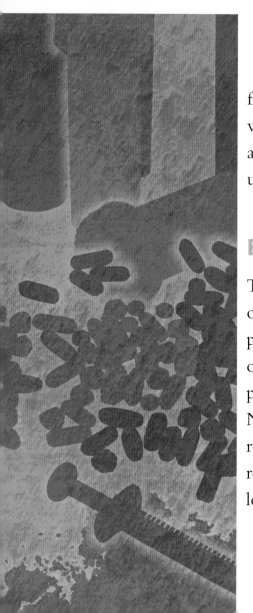

Drug abuse doesn't just ravage your body and mind. It also affects the people around you—your family, friends, and society as a whole. This is a two-way street, however. Americans' attitudes as a society also affect their attitudes toward using drugs.

ENHANCING ONE'S IMAGE

The attitudes of a society have an impact on how people behave. Many Americans place great value on looks and fear getting old. This attitude has a great influence on people's behavior. For example, an Albany, New York, investigation in 2007 and 2008 revealed that a number of celebrities are relying on steroids to keep their bodies looking good, maintain their strength and

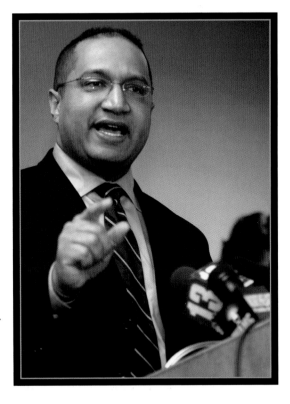

Albany County district attorney David Soares speaks at a news conference, discussing the investigation into a nationwide illegal steroid distribution network.

energy, and fight the effects of aging. According to a January 2008 article in the Albany *Times Union*, stars using steroids include singers, musicians, and actors. The main source of steroids for antiaging applications is doctors who write unjustified prescriptions, often without even seeing the person for whom they are prescribing. The celebrities themselves have not broken any laws because they have obtained the drugs by prescription. However, authorities recently cracked down on a number of "antiaging clinics," facilities that provide therapies to fight the effects of aging. In fact, the organizations targeted by the authorities have been selling millions of dollars' worth of prescription drugs per year, most notably steroids. The stars receive the drugs through the mail from antiaging clinics in New York, Florida, and Texas. In 2007 alone, a number of physicians and managers of such clinics were convicted as a result of the investigation.

47

It's not just celebrities who use steroids to enhance their looks, however. A 2007 study of 1,955 American men who visited online sites related to steroids, published in the *Journal of the International Society of Sports Nutrition*, shows that many of the users of anabolic steroids are highly paid, well-educated professionals who are about thirty years old and are concerned about their looks.

IMPACT ON THE FAMILY

Steroid abuse affects the families of abusers in several ways. First, those who abuse steroids often become more aggressive and violent. Sometimes, they give way to "'roid rage," acts of violent anger. Some studies show that those most likely to become violent when taking steroids are those already prone to be angry and violent.

Even if steroid use doesn't lead to violence, it can ruin a marriage. Steroid abuse can make you inclined to have emotional outbursts and be less able to deal calmly with problems. If a person is married, this behavior can lead to problems between the user and his or her spouse. In addition, a user's spouse often becomes concerned about their children seeing a parent's use of drugs and what effect this will have on them. Also, illegal steroids are expensive, and paying for them may strain the household budget.

Another way in which steroid abuse can hurt the family is through the death of a child or adolescent. Every year, teenagers die as a result of steroid abuse. Sometimes, their deaths are

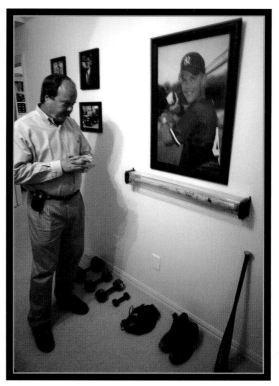

Don Hooton's son, Taylor, committed suicide after using steroids to build muscles. His family and doctors believe that Taylor became very depressed after using the drugs.

accidental. For instance, the steroids they take may over-tax the heart, causing a heart attack. Sometimes, when the steroid use leads to severe depression, teenaged users commit suicide. Either way, the loss of a child has a terrible effect on the family.

THE COSTS TO SOCIETY

The illegal manufacture, sale, and use of steroids have an impact on society in several ways. First, whenever a large number of people use illegal drugs, money is flowing into the hands of criminals. This additional money provides them with the means to engage in even greater criminal activities. Second, studies have shown that when people abuse steroids, they often share needles without sterilizing them in between uses. Viruses that are responsible for serious diseases such as acquired immunodeficiency syndrome (AIDS) and hepatitis are passed from one person to another in the blood. When you inject yourself with a needle, a little of your blood flows back into the needle. When the next person uses the needle, that blood gets injected along with the drug. If you accidentally inject yourself with blood containing a virus for a disease such as AIDS or hepatitis, you can destroy your health. In addition, anything that causes an increase in the number of people who have such serious diseases affects their families as well, and raises health-care costs for society as a whole.

Myths and Facts

Myth: It's a natural substance found in the body, so taking a steroid can't hurt me.

Fact: Natural doesn't mean safe. Many toxic substances occur in nature, but they can damage and even kill you if you take too much.

Myth: Everybody does it, so it's no big deal.

Fact: Everybody doesn't do it. According to the 2007 report by U.S. senator George Mitchell, about 7 percent of professional baseball players rely on steroids. And those who don't would love to see those who do barred from participating.

Myth: Only males use steroids.

Fact: Increasing numbers of women are using steroids to enhance their athletic performance and their looks. According a 2004 study by the U.S. Centers for Disease Control and Prevention, 5.3 percent of girls in grades nine through twelve had used steroids without a prescription.

CHAPTER 6
Steroid Abuse and the Media

Most people know about steroid use through stories they have seen in newspapers and magazines, or on the Internet or TV. Steroid abuse in the media has often been reported in relation to professional sports. On one hand, the media have done the public a service by highlighting the abuse of steroids and showing the negative effects taking steroids can have on users. On the other hand, however, much reporting in the media gives the impression that the use of steroids is so widespread that all players take them. Many people have come to believe that all athletes are cheaters who use steroids, even though this is not true. It might be of benefit to sports and encouraging to young athletes to hear more about athletes who succeed without relying on steroids for their endurance and performance. At one time, young people looked up to sports stars as heroes whom they wished to emulate. Now, they are faced with the choice of copying the bad habits of the present-day crop of players or treating them with contempt.

The media affect steroid use in another way, too. Some people believe that the media hype surrounding professional sports adds to the pressure on athletes to use steroids. The media put great emphasis on breaking records, hitting balls farther, getting greater scores than ever before, and generally outdoing whatever has been done in the past. Breaking records makes great sports news and attracts readers and viewers. Unfortunately, there are limits to what human beings can do naturally. The need to always perform better and better to be thought of as a great athlete could be one factor fueling the use of steroids in sports.

SURFER BEWARE

The Internet is a great place for learning. When you read information on the Web, though, you need to keep a few points in mind. Many people tend to believe that if information is in print, it is fact. This is not necessarily true. There are different types of sites on the Internet. Some sites, like those listed in the back of this book, are run by reputable organizations. They provide information that is vetted and likely to be accurate. A lot of the information on the Web, however, is either inaccurate or personal opinion. In regard to steroid use, you need to

Don't believe everything you read on the Internet. Make sure the information you are seeking comes from a reliable, accurate source. Your parents and teachers can help to recommend reputable sites.

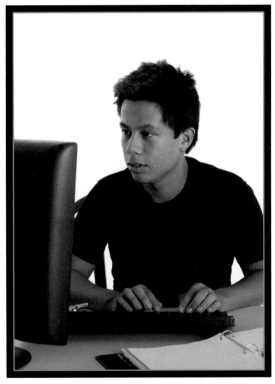

understand that information found on personal Web sites or blogs is just that—personal opinion. When you read that someone has been taking steroids and it's not affecting him or her, this is that person's opinion. It may be a self-serving attempt to justify his or her behavior, the person may not be aware of the toll that the steroid use is taking on his or her body, or the person may even be trying to lure you in to sell you steroids. Therefore, carefully consider the source of any information you read about steroids as you are reading on the Internet.

IT'S UP TO YOU

Now you are equipped with some information about steroids and how they can affect you. Steroids can affect your mental and physical health. If you're caught buying, selling, or using them,

53

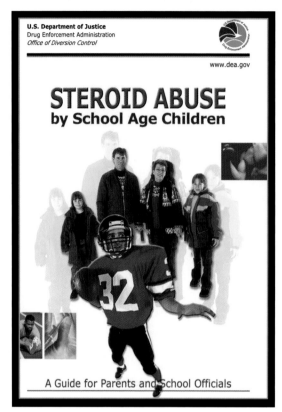

U.S. Department of Justice
Drug Enforcement Administration
Office of Diversion Control

www.dea.gov

STEROID ABUSE
by School Age Children

A Guide for Parents and School Officials

This informative booklet on steroid abuse by young people is available online from the U.S. Department of Justice (www.deadiversion.usdoj.gov). Many government agencies provide online information and publications about drug abuse.

they can affect your future. It's up to you to make an informed decision not to use performance-enhancing drugs. If you refuse to use steroids, you're not alone. A recent study by the University of Michigan shows that steroid use among high school students has been declining over the past several years. Two possible reasons for this decrease are that detection and enforcement procedures have improved, and that young people have become more aware of the health risks. If you are using steroids and want to quit, talk to someone you trust, and get professional help to see you safely through any mental and physical side effects. The more you and your family and friends know about steroids, the more likely you and they will be able to stay away from them.

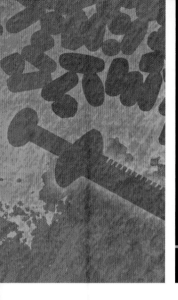

GLOSSARY

adrenal glands Two small glands that are located on the kidneys.

anemia Having too few red blood cells.

autoimmune disease An illness that happens when the body's tissues are attacked by its own immune system.

blog A personal journal a person posts on the Internet for others to read.

cholesterol A fatty substance that can clog arteries.

cut To dilute a drug with another material.

depression An abnormally great feeling of sadness and hopelessness.

hormone A substance that controls an activity in the body.

hypertrophy To grow abnormally large.

inflammation The swelling, redness, heat, and pain that is produced in an area of the body as a reaction to an infection or injury.

manic Frenzied and agitated.

masculinization The development of male characteristics, like facial hair, in women.

megadosing Taking an abnormally large amount of a substance such as steroids.

osteoporosis Loss of bone that occurs as people age.

ovarian cyst A sac that is filled with fluid or a semisolid material and that develops in or on the ovary.

patent medicine A medicine sold without a prescription by a manufacturer. Commonly refers to medicines made and sold in the nineteenth and early twentieth centuries.

physiological Related to body functions.

protein A basic building block of tissue, produced in the body.

psychological Relating to the mind or mental state.

pyramiding Gradually increasing the dose of steroids one takes.

rejuvenate Make a person feel younger.

stacking Taking different forms of steroids or steroids with other drugs at the same time.

sterility Inability to have children.

stroke The clogging of a blood vessel in the brain.

synthetic Man-made.

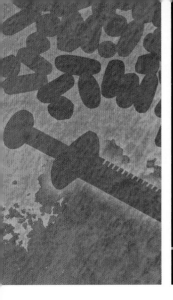

FOR MORE INFORMATION

Canadian Centre on Drug Abuse
75 Albert Street, Suite 300
Ottawa, ON K1P 5E7
Canada
(613) 235-4048
Web site: http://www.ccsa.ca/ccsa
This organization provides a variety of reports and reference materials
on substance abuse in Canada.

Drug Policy Information Clearinghouse
P.O. Box 6000
Rockville, MD 20849-6000
(800) 666-4332
Web site: http://www.whitehousedrugpolicy.org
The Drug Policy Information Clearinghouse provides a wide range of
information on drugs and drug abuse enforcement, treatment, and
prevention, as well as publications.

National Institute on Drug Abuse
National Institutes of Health
6001 Executive Boulevard, Room 5213
Bethesda, MD 20892-9561
(301) 443-1124
Web site: http://www.drugabuse.gov
This organization provides a wealth of information on drug abuse of all types, including steroids, and offers a variety of publications for students and adults.

Substance Abuse and Mental Health Services Administration
1 Choke Cherry Road, Room 8-1036
Rockville, MD 20857
(800) 273-8255
Web site: http://www.samhsa.gov
This agency provides resources to help people recover from substance abuse problems.

WEB SITES

Due to the changing nature of Internet links, Rosen Publishing has developed an online list of Web sites related to the subject of this book. This site is updated regularly. Please use this link to access the list:

http://www.rosenlinks.com/daas/ster

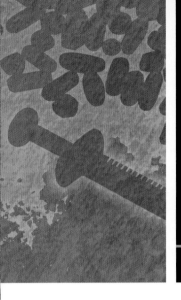

FOR FURTHER READING

Aretha, David. *Steroids and Other Performance-Enhancing Drugs.* Berkeley Heights, NJ: Enslow Publishers, Inc., 2005.

Egendorf, Laura K. *At Issue: Drugs and Sports.* Chicago, IL: Greenhaven Press, 2005.

Fitzhugh, Karla. *Health Issues: Steroids.* Chicago, IL: Raintree, 2003.

Lau, Doretta. *Steroids* (Incredibly Disgusting Drugs). New York, NY: Rosen Publishing, 2008.

LeVert, Suzanne. *The Truth About Steroids.* New York, NY: Benchmark Books, 2004.

Lukas, Scott E. *The Drug Library: Steroids.* Berkeley Heights, NJ: Enslow Publishers, Inc., 2001.

Mintzer, Richard. *Steroids = Busted!* Berkeley Heights, NJ: Enslow Publishers, Inc., 2006.

Monroe, Judy. *Steroids, Sports, and Body Image: The Risks of Performance-Enhancing Drugs.* Berkeley Heights, NJ: Enslow Publishers, Inc., 2004.

Walker, Ida. *Steroids: Pumped Up and Dangerous.* Broomall, PA: Mason Crest Publishers, 2007.

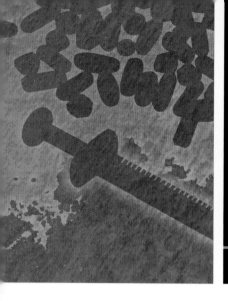

BIBLIOGRAPHY

Association Against Steroid Use. "Coming Off Anabolic Steroids." Retrieved January 22, 2008 (http://www.steroidabuse.com/coming-off-steroids.html).

Cohen, Jason, Rick Collins, Jack Darkes, and Daniel Gwartney. "A League of Their Own: Demographics, Motivations and Patterns of Use of 1,955 Male Adult Non-medical Anabolic Steroid Users in the United States." *Journal of the International Society of Sports Nutrition*, Vol. 4 No. 12, 2007. Retrieved January 25, 2008 (http://www.jissn.com/content/4/1/12).

International Herald Tribune. "Jones Gets 6-Month Prison Term for Steroids and Fraud Scam." January 11, 2008. Retrieved January 21, 2008 (http://www.iht.com/articles/2008/01/11/sports/doping.php).

Jendrick, Nathan. *Dunks, Doubles, Doping: How Steroids Are Killing American Athletics.* Guilford, CT: The Lyons Press, 2006.

Johnston, L. D., P. M. O'Malley, J. G. Bachman, and J. E. Schulenberg. *Monitoring the Future. National Results on Adolescent Drug Use: Overview of Key Findings, 2007.* Bethesda, MD:

National Institute on Drug Abuse, 2008. Retrieved March 4, 2008 (http://www.monitoringthefuture.org/data/07data/fig07_13.pdf).

Laos, Carla, and Jordan D. Metzl. "Performance-Enhancing Drug Use in Young Athletes." *Adolescent Medicine*, Vol. 17, 2006, pp. 719–731.

Lyons, Brendan J. "Steroids Beyond Sports." *Times Union* (Albany, NY), January 13, 2008. Retrieved January 14, 2008 (http://timesunion.com/ASPStories/storyPrint.asp?StoryID=654817).

Mitchell, George J. *Report to the Commissioner of Baseball of an Independent Investigation into the Illegal Use of Steroids and Other Performance-Enhancing Substances by Players in Major League Baseball*. December 13, 2007. Retrieved December 13, 2007 (http://files.mlb.com/mitchrpt.pdf).

National Institute on Drug Abuse. "NIDA InfoFacts: Steroids (Anabolic-Androgenic)." National Institutes of Health. Retrieved January 2, 2008 (http://www.drugabuse.gov/Infofacts/steroids.html).

Snow, Chris, and Gordon Edes. "Former Sox Starter Admits Steroid Use." *Boston Globe*, June 22, 2006. Retrieved January 21, 2007 (http://www.boston.com/sports/baseball/redsox/articles/2006/06/22/former_sox_starter_admits_steroid_use).

USA Today. "BALCO Investigation Timeline." Retrieved January 25, 2008 (http://www.usatoday.com/sports/balco-timeline.htm).

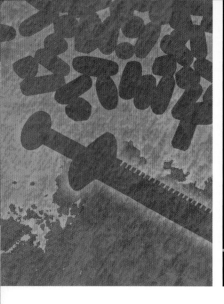

INDEX

L

Lorz, Fred, 9–10

M

masculinization, 13, 25
megadosing, 20
Mitchell, George, 41–42, 50
Mitchell Report, 41–43
Monitoring the Future survey, 2007, 15

N

needle sharing, dangers of, 49–50

O

Organon Company, 9

P

peer pressure, 22
performance-enhancing substances, history
    of, 9–12
pyramiding, 20

R

rehabilitation centers, 33
Ruzicka, Leopold, 9

S

Schering Corporation, 9
stacking, 21
Steinach, Eugen, 8
sterility/ability to have children, 24, 25
steroids
    discovery of, 7–9
    explanation of, 4–6
    how they work, 14–15
    and major league sports/professional ath-
        letes, 4, 7, 12, 40–45, 52
    medical uses of, 5, 6, 16
    and the Olympics, 10–12, 13, 45
    physical effects of abuse of, 23–25
    psychological effects of abuse of, 26
    statistics, 15
    why people use, 5–6, 16–17, 29–31
    withdrawal symptoms, 35–36

T

testosterone, 4–5, 8, 9, 12, 24, 25, 26

U

U.S. Drug Enforcement Administration, 38

ABOUT THE AUTHOR

Jeri Freedman earned a B.A. degree from Harvard University. For fifteen years, she worked for companies in the medical field. Among the numerous books she has written for young adults are *Hemophilia, Hepatitis B, Lymphoma: Current and Emerging Trends in Detection and Treatment, How Do We Know About Genetics and Heredity?, The Mental and Physical Effects of Obesity, Everything You Need to Know About Genetically Modified Foods, Autism,* and *Tay-Sachs Disease.*

PHOTO CREDITS

Pp. 5, 19, 38, 54 U.S. Drug Enforcement Administration; p. 8 © Roger-Viollet/The Image Works; p. 11 John Dominis/Time & Life Pictures/Getty Images; p. 13 © Alfred Pasieka/Photo Researchers, Inc.; pp. 14, 21 Shutterstock.com; p. 23 © Dr. P. Marazzi/Photo Researchers, Inc.; p. 24 © Lauren Shear/Photo Researchers, Inc.; p. 30 © www.istockphoto.com/Gary Milner; p. 32 © www.istockphoto.com/Bart Coenders; p. 35 © www.istockphoto.com/Sheryl Griffin; p. 41 © Tim Sloan/AFP/Getty Images; p. 44 © Don Emmert/AFP/Getty Images; pp. 47, 49 © AP Images; p. 53 © www.istockphoto.com/Ana Abejon.

Designer: Tahara Anderson; Editor: Kathy Kuhtz Campbell